SPECTACULAR NAIL ART

A Step-by-Step Guide to 35 Gorgeous Designs

LARIT LEVY

Photography by Roee Fainburg

imagine!

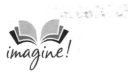
imagine!

An Imagine Book
Published by Charlesbridge
85 Main Street, Watertown, MA 02472
617-926-0329
www.charlesbridge.com

Created by Penn Publishing Ltd.
1 Yehuda Halevi Street, Tel Aviv, Israel 65135
www.penn.co.il

Editor-in-Chief: Rachel Penn
Edited by Shoshana Brickman
Photography by Roee Fainburg
Design and layout by Ariane Rybski

Library of Congress Cataloging-in-Publication Data

Levy, Larit.
Spectacular nail art : a step-by-step guide to 35 gorgeous designs / Larit Levy ; photography by Roee Fainburg.
    pages cm
"An Imagine Book."
Includes bibliographical references.
ISBN 978-1-62354-025-8 (alk. paper)
1. Nail art (Manicuring) I. Title.
TT958.3.L48 2013
646.7'27--dc23
                              2013017629

2 4 6 8 10 9 7 5 3 1

Printed in China, September 2013

For information about custom editions, special sales, premium and corporate purchases, please contact
Charlesbridge Publishing at specialsales@charlesbridge.com

TABLE OF CONTENTS

BASICS

Introduction

Manicures, nail polish and the wonders of nail art are a world unto themselves these days. There are so many amazing shades of nail polish and no end to the types of nail products available on the internet and in nail shops. Nail art can suit any type occasion and style, from high-end affairs to casual street looks. All you need are simple tools and materials, practice and inspiration.

Inspiration is exactly where *Spectacular Nail Art* fits in. You'll find 35 colorful ideas to help you to create awesome nail art with ease. Whether you're preparing for a special occasion or simply want to liven up your everyday look, you'll find something that fits the bill right here. Every project includes easy-to-follow instructions and step-by-step photos.

As with all things in life, patience pays off when it comes to nail art. If you're a beginner, things may take a bit longer than you expect, but don't be discouraged. After a while, the process gets easier and the results become more impressive. And remember – enjoy yourself. Because really, that's the most important thing!

Caring for Your Hands and Nails

Here are some tips to keep your hands and nails healthy and beautiful:

➲ Always wear gloves when you use cleaning products.

➲ Dry your hands thoroughly after washing them, and then apply moisturizing cream. Rub the cream into your hands, especially in the area around the nails, until it is completely absorbed.

➲ If you suffer from dry or hard skin around your nails, rub cuticle oil into the area every day, massaging it in thoroughly.

➲ Always use acetone-free nail polish remover to remove nail polish.

➲ File your nails with emery boards made from natural materials such as paper or cardboard. Don't use metallic boards, as these are likely to do more harm than good.

➲ When caring for the skin around your nails, use a cuticle stick made from natural materials such as an orange-wood cuticle stick. Never use a metal cuticle stick, as this can damage both your nails and the skin around them.

➲ When choosing a nail salon, select one that is hygienic and uses treatments that are gentle on your skin. If the salon is not sterile or the treatment is too rough, it could damage your skin or cause bacterial infections.

➲ Don't use callus shavers to remove tough or hardened skin, as this can damage the skin and ultimately lead to even tougher skin.

➲ Avoid nail salons that use machines to dry the nail polish, as this can cause dry skin which leads to premature skin aging and other problems.

MATERIALS

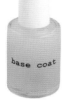

Base coat

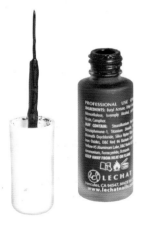

Dotting tool

French manicure kit

Base coat
This transparent polish is applied to nails before colored polish to prevent the colored polish from entering the pigment.

Cotton balls or pads
Use these to apply nail polish remover. If you don't have any on hand, you can also use paper towels or tissues.

Dotting tools
These are designed especially for making dots, but can be used to achieve all sorts of amazing designs. Dotting tools are sold at nail supply stores and online but you can also make dotting tools at home. To make a tool for creating medium-sized dots, insert the sharp end of a head pin into the eraser of a pencil. To make a tool for larger dots, use the tip of an ordinary pen. To make small dots, a toothpick can usually do the trick.

French manicure kit
These are sold in most places that sell nail polish and supplies. The nail polish usually comes with a long thin brush that's perfect for creating the tip of the French manicure. This brush is also great for drawing nail art designs.

Nail art brush
Use this to draw lines, dots, and other fine details on your nails. Choose one that is comfortable to use and of good quality so that the bristles don't get ruined (or ruin your design). Clean the brush thoroughly after every use, or when you switch colors within a single design. To do this, first wipe the brush with a cotton ball or pad and then dip it in nail polish remover. Wipe the brush again to make sure it is clean.

Nail polish
Always choose high-quality nail polish, since it is more durable. After all, considering the time and effort you've put into creating your nail art, you want it to last for a long time! Also, high-quality nail polish usually comes with a good brush, which makes it easier to apply the polish smoothly. The nail polish colors used in this book are for inspiration only. Add, change or vary the colors as much as you like.

Nail polish remover
Don't even start polishing your nails without first making sure that you have nail polish remover on hand. Not only will you need it to clean brushes and dotting tools, but you'll also need it to remove old nail polish. Keep the remover close at hand while applying nail polish, as you may need it to remove some as you go should anything look not quite right. Always use acetone-free nail polish remover.

Stickers and adhesive tape

These are used to create nail designs that require a level of precision that is hard to achieve using nail polish brushes. A few designs in this book require adhesive tape, round stickers and extra-thin nail stickers.

Toothpicks

These can be used instead of a dotting tool to make small dots or draw delicate lines.

Top coat

This transparent polish speeds up the drying process of the nail polish and protects nail polish from chipping. Most top coats also add shine, although there are also varieties that leave a matte finish. I recommend waiting for about 15 to 30 minutes before applying top coat to nail art that includes details. This allows the details to dry thoroughly and prevents them from being accidentally smudged. To keep polished nails looking shiny and fresh, apply a top coat every day.

| Adhesive tape | Extra-thin nail sticker | Round stickers | Toothpicks | Top coat |

TECHNIQUES

How to Do a Manicure at Home

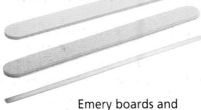

Emery boards and
orange-wood cuticle stick

It's time-consuming (and expensive!) to go to a nail salon regularly, so learning how to care for your hands and nails at home is important. Although I recommend having a professional remove dry or dead skin around nails, all other elements of hand and nail care can be taken care of at home.

1. File your nails into a shape you like – round, oval, square or 'squoval'. Never file your nails too short as this can be painful and damage the skin. Make sure your nails are dry when you file them. Although professionals often file nails when they are wet, soaking nails in advance causes them to expand and this makes the shaping process difficult to control.
2. Apply moisturizing cream to your hands and rub it in thoroughly.
3. Rub cuticle cream into the skin around each nail and massage it in thoroughly.
4. Prepare a bowl of warm water with bath salts or another gentle cleansing material. Don't use soap as this will cause your hands to dry out.

5. Soak your hands in the warm water for a few minutes and then dry them gently with a towel. Use an orange-wood cuticle stick to gently push back any skin that is on the nails. Don't push back skin that is at the base of the nail; just push back skin that's on the nail.
6. Dry your hands and nails thoroughly and then apply a thin base coat to the nails.
7. Let the base coat dry for about 30 seconds and then apply a coat of nail polish. Let the nail polish dry for about 30 seconds and then apply a second coat.
8. Let the nail polish dry for about 2 or 3 minutes and then apply a top coat.

How to Apply Nail Polish

You can get great results from a home manicure with a bit of patience and a lot of practice.

1. Make sure your nails are completely clean and don't have any traces of old nail polish.
2. Apply a transparent base coat first. To apply the base coat, dip the polish brush into the base coat and then draw the brush against the inside of the bottle opening to avoid having too much polish on the brush. You want enough polish to make a few strokes on the nail, but not so much polish that it drips off the brush.
3. Start by applying the nail polish at the middle base of the nail. Place the brush on the nail at the cuticle and draw it to the tip of the nail in a single smooth motion.
4. After painting a single strip along the middle of the nail, place the brush back at the cuticle, to one side of the middle strip, and draw it to the tip of the nail in a single smooth motion. Repeat again on the other side of the middle strip.
5. Continue applying the polish in strips, from the base to the tip, until the entire nail is covered. Dip the brush into the nail polish as required.
6. Repeat this process to apply a base coat to all the nails and then let the base coat dry for about 30 seconds.
7. Hold the bottle of nail polish you'll be using and roll it gently between your hands to mix the nail polish so that the color is homogenous. Don't shake the bottle since you don't want any bubbles to form.
8. Open the bottle and draw the nail polish brush against the inside of the bottle opening just like you did with the base coat.
9. As before, start by applying the nail polish at the middle base of the nail. Place the brush on the nail at the cuticle and draw it to the tip of the nail in a single smooth motion. Continue applying nail polish on both sides of the middle strip until the entire nail is covered. Repeat this process on all the nails. Each nail should be covered with a single, relatively light layer of nail polish. Try to get as close to the base of the nail without painting on the skin. Nail

polish that starts on the skin rather than the nail chips faster and doesn't look great, either.

10. Apply a second layer of nail polish in the same manner as the first layer, until the color is smooth and consistent. If the polish isn't as thick or smooth as you'd like, apply a third layer of nail polish.

11. Wait for about 2 or 3 minutes to let the polish dry, and then apply top coat in a similar manner to seal the color and prevent the polish from chipping.

How to Do a French Manicure

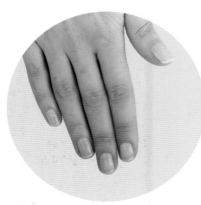

Before a French Manicure

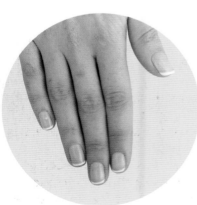

After a French Manicure

A French manicure is a classic manicure in which the nail polish is applied in a manner that mimics the nails' natural appearance. Usually, a natural-colored pink, beige or transparent base polish is applied first and then the tip of the nail is painted white.

French manicures are popular all over the world, and probably have been since the 1920s or 30s. While the standard version involves a pink base and opaque white tips, there are many alternatives today. American manicures, for example, use a beige base rather than a pink one. For a more natural look, try painting the tips with pearly white nail polish rather than stark white nail polish. You can also use completely non-traditional color combinations, such as red nails with white tips or pink nails with black tips.

1. Apply a base coat and let it dry. Apply two coats of transparent or opaque light pink or beige nail polish and let it dry.

2. Dip a thin nail art brush into the white nail polish, and place it in the middle of the nail, at the place where the nail tip naturally starts. Draw a line to the left edge of the nail.

3. Pick up the brush and place it back at the middle of the nail. Draw it across the nail in the other direction, to make a line to the right edge of the nail.

4. Continue applying white nail polish, from the line you just painted to the tip of the nail, until this area is completely filled.

5. Let the polish dry for about 2 to 3 minutes and then apply a top coat.

TIPS

➲ You can also try painting the white tips first and then applying transparent pink or beige nail polish over the entire nail. This softens the brightness of the white tips and creates a more natural look.

➲ Regarding the shape and width of the white strip at the top of the nail, I recommend basing this on the natural shape and location of the nail tip. When painting particularly long nails, soften the look by using milky white, rather than opaque white, nail polish for the tip.

How to Use a Dotting Tool

Using a dotting tool is easy and quite fun. Simply dip the tool into the nail polish and then place it on the nail. You'll have to work quickly so that the nail polish doesn't dry before it reaches the nail. If it does, simply dip the tool into the polish again.

If you've got a lot of dotting to do, I suggest that you pour a little mound of nail polish onto a piece of cardboard or plastic and dip the tool into this, since this makes the process easier and quicker. If you are only making a few dots, dip the dotting tool directly into the bottle of nail polish. If you do it this way, make sure you close the bottle immediately after dipping so that the polish in the bottle doesn't dry out.

Small mounds of nail polish for making dots

How to Use Stickers and Adhesive Tape

The first few times you use stickers or tape to create nail art will probably be quite frustrating. The technique requires a bit of skill and a lot of patience. Here are some tips to help speed up the learning process (and hopefully reduce the amount of angry whispering you do under your breath):

1. Apply the nail polish that will be the base for the design in really thin coats, and then let it dry for at least 30 minutes. This helps prevent the polish from peeling off when you remove the sticker.
2. Before placing the sticker on the nail, put the sticky side of it on your hand and gently pull it off to make it less sticky. This reduces the chance that your sticker will peel off the base nail polish when it is removed. Repeat this process a few times.
3. Place the sticker on the nail and then apply the nail polish. Let the polish dry for 30 to 60 seconds before peeling off the sticker. Don't wait too long to remove the sticker because if the polish is too dry, it will be rubbery when you pull off the sticker and might leave stretchy strings of polish. If the nail polish is too wet when you remove the sticker, you might smear the design.
4. Peel off the sticker in a single, gentle pull backwards – not upwards. This may be the trickiest part of the whole process, so be patient (and good luck)!

CHAMPAGNE CHIC

With this sparkling design, you'll look fantastic holding
a glass of bubbly at midnight.

MATERIALS

For the Base:
- Black nail polish

For the Design:
- Gold nail polish

TOOLS
- Small dotting tool

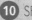

STEP 1

Apply a base coat to the nails and let it dry. Apply two coats of black nail polish and let it dry completely.

STEP 2

Dip the small dotting tool into the gold nail polish and make a line of dots along the top edge of the tip of the nail. Place the dots really close together and really close to the edge.

STEP 3

Make another row of dots immediately below the first row. These dots should also be really close together.

STEP 4

Make two more rows of dots below the second one, leaving more space between each dot.

STEP 5

Place a few dots on the rest of the nail, in a scattered fashion. Make sure these dots are not too close together. Repeat these steps on the rest of the nails to create a bubbling champagne effect.

TIPS

• Wait until the polish is completely dry and then apply a top coat to seal and protect the design.
• Refresh the top coat regularly to keep the design looking fresh.

POSITIVELY PATRIOTIC

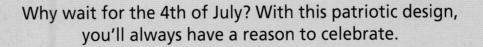

Why wait for the 4th of July? With this patriotic design,
you'll always have a reason to celebrate.

MATERIALS

For the Base:
- Red nail polish
- Metallic blue nail polish

For the Design:
- Opaque white nail polish

TOOLS
- Thin nail art brush
- Medium dotting tool

STEP 1

Apply a base coat to the nails and let it dry. Apply two coats of red nail polish to four nails, leaving the nail on the ring finger bare. Let the polish dry.

STEP 2

Dip the thin nail art brush into the opaque white nail polish and draw a thick horizontal line across the bottom of the nail. Leave a thick strip of red nail polish visible at the base of the nail. Repeat this step, if necessary, to make a line with substance.

STEP 3

Repeat this process a few more times to create three or four horizontal lines across the nail.

The actual number of lines you draw on each nail depends on the length of the nail. Try to make sure that the space you leave between each line is similar to the width of the line. Repeat these steps on the rest of the nails that have been painted with red polish.

STEP 4

Apply two coats of metallic blue nail polish on the ring finger nail and let the polish dry.

STEP 5

Dip the dotting tool into the opaque white nail polish and make several dots on the blue nail. Make sure the dots are evenly spaced.

TIPS

• Wait until the nail polish is completely dry and then apply a top coat to seal and protect the design. Refresh the top coat regularly to keep the design looking fresh.
• To make horizontal lines that are thick and straight, place the tip of the brush at one edge of the nail and then rotate the nail towards the brush.

SNAPPY SNOWFLAKES

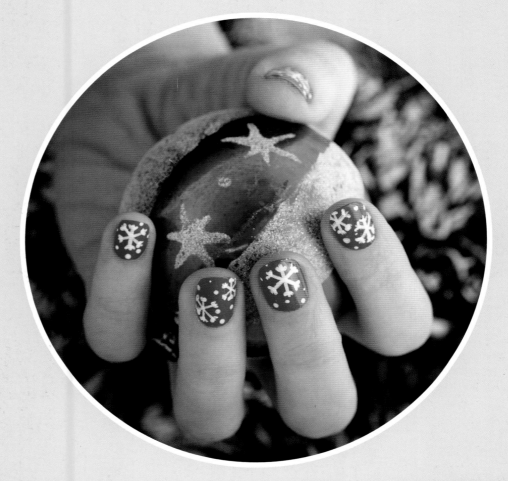

No need for cold weather to enjoy a snowy Christmas. With this design, you can have flakes whenever you want!

MATERIALS

For the Base:
• Red nail polish

For the Design:
• Opaque white nail polish

TOOLS
• Thin nail art brush
• Dotting tool

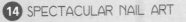

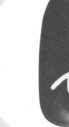

1

2

4

5

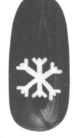

6

STEP 1

Apply a base coat to the nails and let it dry. Apply two coats of red nail polish and let it dry completely. Plan where you want to position the snowflake and decide where the center of that snowflake will be. Dip the thin nail art brush into the opaque white nail polish and place it at this point. Make a small thin line that starts here and extends in any direction.

STEP 2

Place the brush at the beginning of the line you just made and draw a similar line at a 30° angle to the first line. This line should be the same length as the first line.

STEP 3

Repeat this process four more times to make a 6-branch star on the nail. Try to make the lines evenly spaced and of the same length.

STEP 4

Now draw a pair of tiny branches very close to the tip of one of these branches, to make a tiny 3-pronged tip.

STEP 5

Repeat this step to make 3-pronged tips on the end of each branch.

STEP 6

Dip the dotting tool into the opaque white nail polish and make scattered dots all over the nail. Repeat this process to make snowflakes on all the nails. If you like, make two snowflakes on the larger nails.

TIPS

• Wait until the polish is completely dry and then apply a top coat to seal and protect the design.
• Refresh the top coat regularly to keep the design looking fresh.

JOLLY SANTA

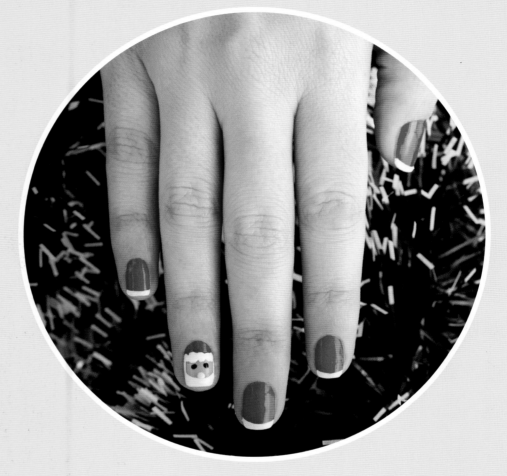

Bring out the Santa in your heart with this jolly design.

MATERIALS

For the Base:
• Red nail polish

For the Design:
• Opaque white nail polish
• Black nail polish
• Pink nail polish

TOOLS

• Dotting tool
• Thin nail art brush

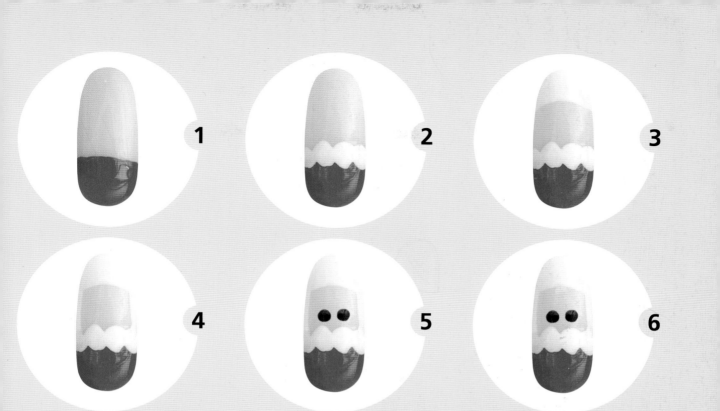

STEP 1
Apply a base coat to the nails and let it dry. Apply two coats of red nail polish to the bottom third of the ring finger nail (near the base) and let it dry completely. Leave the top two-thirds of the nail bare.

STEP 2
Dip the dotting tool into the opaque white nail polish and make a crowded row of white dots along the edge of the red nail polish to 'soften' the edge. This will be the bottom of Santa's hat.

STEP 3
Dip the thin nail art brush into the opaque white nail polish and draw a thick line along the tip of the nail. This will be Santa's beard.

STEP 4
Still using the thin nail art brush, draw lines along the sides of the nail, from the bottom of the hat to the beard. These will be Santa's sideburns. Make the lines as thick as necessary, depending upon the width of the nail.

STEP 5
Dip the dotting tool into the black nail polish and make two dots below the white edge of Santa's hat, for eyes.

STEP 6
Clean the dotting tool thoroughly and then dip it into the pink nail polish and make a dot for the nose. Wait until the polish is

completely dry and then apply a top coat to seal and protect the design.

STEP 7
Apply two coats of red nail polish to the rest of the nails and let the polish dry. Dip the thin nail art brush into the opaque white nail polish and draw a thick strip of white across the tip of each nail. Apply a second coat of white polish to make the tips bright. Let the polish dry for about 2 to 3 minutes and then apply a top coat.

TIP
Refresh the top coat regularly to keep the design looking fresh.

COBWEBBY CREATIONS

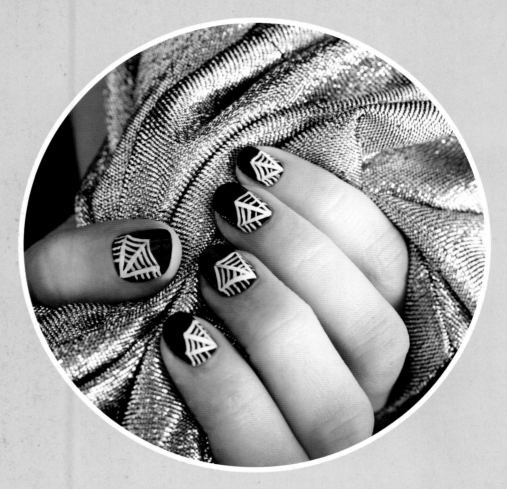

Extend your Halloween décor right to your fingertips with stunning spidery design.

MATERIALS

For the Base:
- Black nail polish

For the Design:
- Opaque white nail polish

TOOLS
- Thin nail art brush

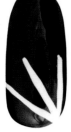
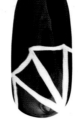
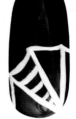

3

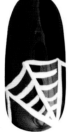

4

5

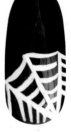

6

STEP 1

Apply a base coat to the nails and let it dry. Apply two coats of black nail polish and let it dry completely. Dip the thin nail art brush into the opaque white nail polish and draw a line from one corner of the nail at the base towards the middle of the nail. Draw another line, starting at the same place and of the same length, at a 30° angle above this line. Now draw a third line, starting at the same place and of the same length, at a 30° angle below the first line.

STEP 2

Draw a curved line between the tip of the rightmost line and the tip of the middle line to create a triangular shape. Draw another curved line between the tip of the middle line and the tip of the leftmost line. Draw two more curved lines, one extending from the leftmost line to the left edge of the nail, and the other extending from the rightmost line to the right edge of the nail.

STEP 3

Make several evenly spaced curved lines inside one of the triangular shapes that you made in step 2.

STEP 4

Repeat this process with the other triangular shape that you made in step 2 to create the appearance of a web.

STEP 5

Repeat this process again from the leftmost outer line to the left edge of the nail.

STEP 6

Repeat this process again from the rightmost outer line to the right edge of the nail.

TIPS

• Wait until the polish is completely dry and then apply a top coat to seal and protect the design.
• Refresh the top coat regularly to keep the design looking fresh.

POSITIVELY PUMPKIN

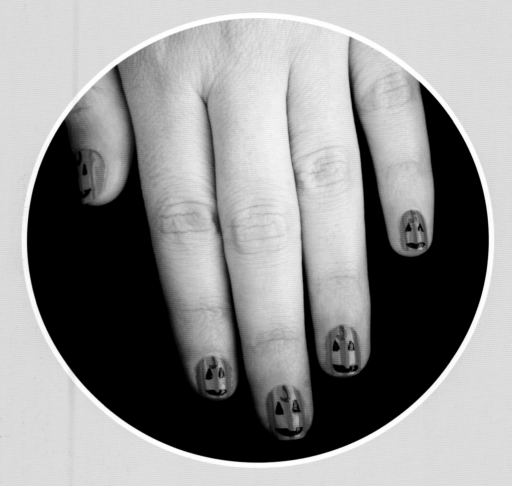

These perky pumpkins require absolutely no carving!

MATERIALS

For the Base:
- Orange nail polish

For the Design:
- Red nail polish
- Black nail polish
- Green nail polish

TOOLS
- Thin nail art brush
- Toothpick

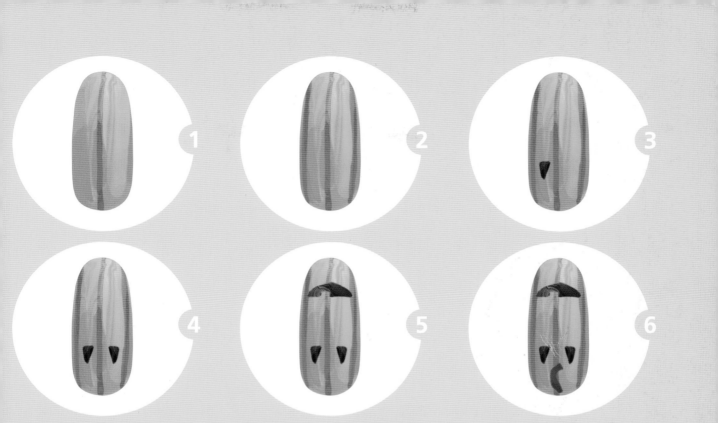

STEP 1

Apply a base coat to the nails and let it dry. Apply two coats of orange nail polish and let it dry completely. Dip the thin nail art brush into the red nail polish and draw a vertical line, from the base of the nail to the tip, down the middle of the nail.

STEP 2

Draw two more lines, one on either side of the middle line, and at even distances from it.

STEP 3

Dip a toothpick into the black nail polish and draw a small triangle with the tip towards the base of the nail on the left side of the nail, between two red lines, to make an eye.

STEP 4

Make a similar triangle on the right side of the nail to make the other eye.

STEP 5

Still using a toothpick, draw a semi-circle with an upwards curve near the tip of the nail for the mouth. Draw a line with a square-shaped detour near the middle connecting the two ends of the semicircle. Fill in the space between the two lines with black nail polish to give the appearance of an open mouth with a single tooth.

STEP 6

Clean the toothpick thoroughly (or simply get a new one) and dip it into the green nail polish. Draw

a little curved line at the base of the nail, to create the stem. Repeat this process to make perky pumpkins on all the nails.

TIPS

• Wait until the polish is completely dry and then apply a top coat to seal and protect the design.
• Refresh the top coat regularly to keep the design looking fresh.

SPARKLY HEART

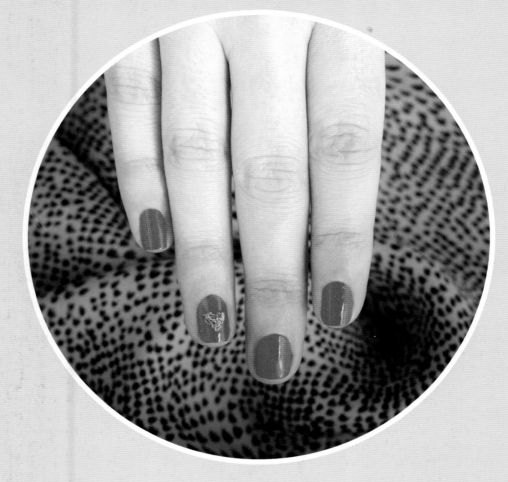

This simple sparkly design says "Love, Love, Love!" Perfect for Valentine's Day.

MATERIALS

For the Base:

• Fuchsia nail polish

For the Design:

• Sparkly silver nail polish

TOOLS

• Adhesive tape

• Scissors

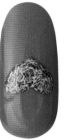

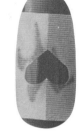

STEP 1
Apply a base coat to the nails and let it dry. Apply two coats of fuchsia nail polish and let it dry completely.

STEP 2
Place a 2-inch piece of adhesive tap on your hand (not yet on your nail) and pull it off. Repeat this action a few times to reduce the stickiness of the tape, and then fold the tape in half, sticky sides facing. Cut a tiny half-heart shape at the fold so that when you unfold the tape, you get a full heart. Unfold the tape to see that the heart shape you created is just right. Make sure the nail polish has dried completely and then place the tape with the cut-out heart onto the ring finger nail, so that the heart space is in the center of the nail.

STEP 3
Paint a thick layer of sparkly silver nail polish on the heart-shaped area that's been cut out of the tape. Don't worry about getting nail polish on the edges of the tape because you'll be removing it anyway.

STEP 4
Let the nail polish dry for about 30 seconds and then gently remove the tape, peeling it away backwards, rather than upwards, so that the nail polish doesn't smudge. Repeat steps 2 and 3 to draw a heart on the ring finger nail of the other hand.

TIPS
• Wait until the polish is completely dry and then apply a top coat to seal and protect the design.
• Refresh the top coat regularly to keep the design looking fresh.
• For tips on using adhesive tape, see page 9.

VINTAGE FLOWERS

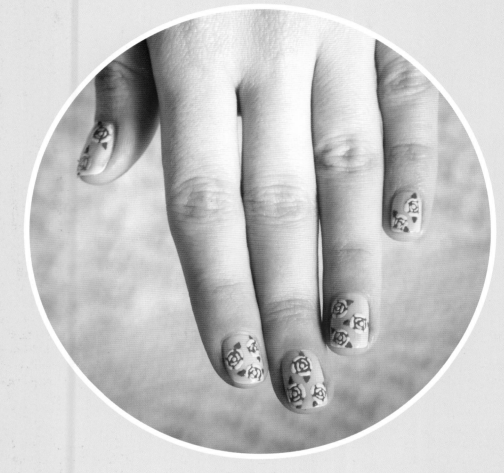

Evoke the grandeur of your grandma's favorite sofa with this fancy floral design.

MATERIALS

For the Base:
- Very light pink nail polish

For the Design:
- Fuchsia nail polish
- Light pink nail polish
- Green nail polish

TOOLS
- Toothpick

STEP 1

Apply a base coat to the nails and let it dry. Apply two coats of very light pink nail polish and let it dry completely. Apply a third coat, if necessary, so that the polish is homogenous. Dip the tip of the nail polish brush into the fuchsia nail polish and make a few large dots on the nail. Don't worry about making the shape of the dots perfectly round. Let the polish dry.

STEP 2

Dip a toothpick into the light pink nail polish and draw a dashed line, made up of 3 or 4 dashes, around the edge of one of the fuchsia dots. You'll have to dab the toothpick onto the nail to make this line rather than draw it a single smooth motion.

STEP 3

Repeat this step to draw dashed lines around all of the fuchsia dots. If you find that the nail polish builds up on the toothpick, wipe it clean with a cotton ball dipped in nail polish remover.

STEP 4

Still using the toothpick, make a light pink dot in the middle of each fuchsia dot.

STEP 5

Continue using a toothpick to draw little curved lines around the light pink dot in the middle of each fuchsia dot, to make petals.

STEP 6

Clean the toothpick (or simply use a new one) and dip it in the green

nail polish. Draw tiny triangular leaves on either side of each flower. Place the leaves at different locations for each flower. Repeat these steps to draw flowers on every nail.

TIPS

• If you like, place the flowers at different locations on each nail.
• Wait until the polish is completely dry and then apply a top coat to seal and protect the design.
• Refresh the top coat regularly to keep the design looking fresh.

HAWAIIAN HIBISCUS

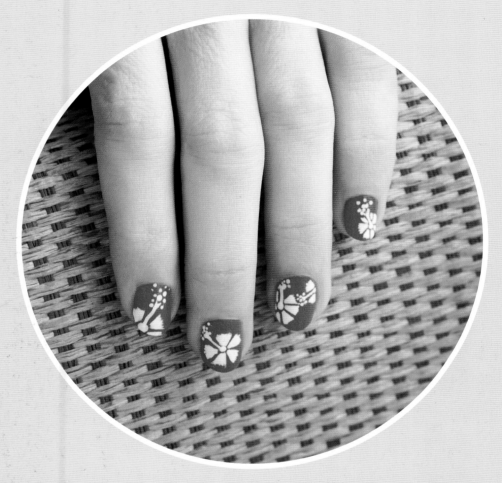

Consider yourself warned: this design has been know to cause an immediate urge for a Hawaiian holiday!

MATERIALS

For the Base:
- Fuchsia nail polish

For the Design:
- Opaque white nail polish

TOOLS
- Thin nail art brush
- Toothpick or small dotting tool

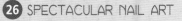

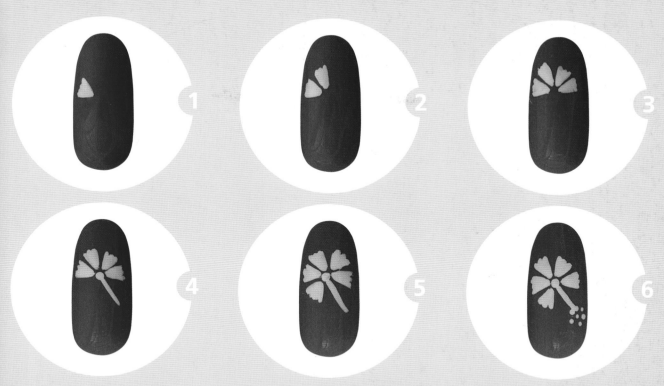

STEP 1
Apply a base coat to the nails and let it dry. Apply two coats of fuchsia nail polish and let it dry completely. Dip the thin nail art brush into the opaque white nail polish and then press the side of the brush onto the nail, near one edge but not touching it, to make a tiny wedge shape. Repeat this process two more times, rotating the bristles of the brush just a bit, to make a triangular flower petal with a wavy edge.

STEP 2
Repeat this process to make a second petal close to the first one. Be sure to leave a strip of fuchsia nail polish showing between the two petals.

STEP 3
Repeat this process again to make two more petals.

STEP 4
Dip the small dotting tool or toothpick into the opaque white nail polish and draw a small dot in the middle of all four petals. Draw a thin line extending from the dot. This is the flower's pistil.

STEP 5
Using the thin nail art brush again, draw one more petal to complete the flower.

STEP 6
Using the small dotting tool or toothpick and the opaque white nail polish, draw a tiny horizontal line at the tip of the pistil and then draw several small dots, to create the pollen. Repeat these steps to draw flowers on every nail.

TIPS
• If you like, place the flowers at different places on each nail.
• Wait until the polish is completely dry and then apply a top coat to seal and protect the design.
• Refresh the top coat regularly to keep the design looking fresh.
• If there is room, you can draw two flowers on a nail.

DARLIN' DAISIES

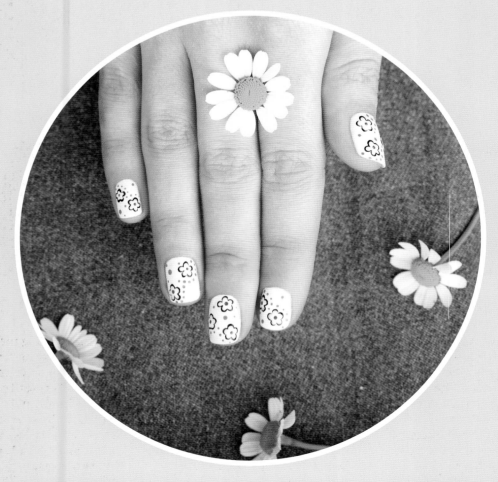

These gorgeous flowers are as much fun to make as they are to wear—like an all-day bouquet on your hands.

MATERIALS

For the Base:
- Opaque white nail polish

For the Design:
- Black nail polish
- Fuchsia nail polish
- Turquoise nail polish

TOOLS

- Medium dotting tool
- Small dotting tool or toothpick

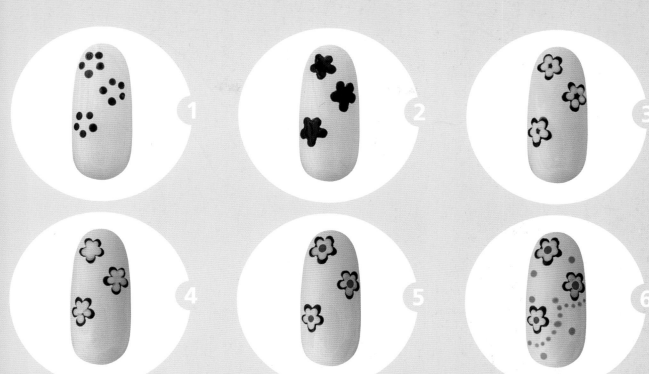

STEP 1

Apply a base coat to the nails and let it dry. Apply two coats of opaque white nail polish and let it dry completely. Dip the medium dotting tool into the black nail polish and make three clusters of five dots on the nail. These dots will be the flower petals, so arrange them accordingly. As for the number of clusters, you can make more if there is room on the nail.

STEP 2

Dip the dotting tool back into the nail polish and fill in the spaces between the dots, to make flowers.

STEP 3

Clean the dotting tool thoroughly and then dip it into the white nail polish. Make five dots on each flower to make a smaller white flower on top of the larger black flower.

STEP 4

Dip the dotting tool back into the white nail polish and fill in the spaces between the dots.

STEP 5

Clean the dotting tool thoroughly and then dip it into the fuchsia nail polish. Make a single dot in the center of each flower.

STEP 6

Clean the dotting tool again and dip it into the turquoise nail polish. Make some scattered dots in the white space between the flowers. Use both the small and medium dotting tools to make a diagonal line of small and medium dots across the middle of the nail. Repeat these steps to make pretty daisy designs on all the nails.

TIPS

• Wait until the nails are completely dry and then apply a top coat to seal and protect the design.
• Refresh the top coat regularly to keep the design looking fresh.

LADYBUG LUCK

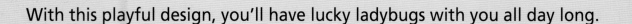

With this playful design, you'll have lucky ladybugs with you all day long.

MATERIALS

For the Base:
- Red nail polish

For the Design:
- Black nail polish
- Opaque white nail polish

TOOLS
- Thin nail art brush
- Large dotting tool
- Small dotting tool

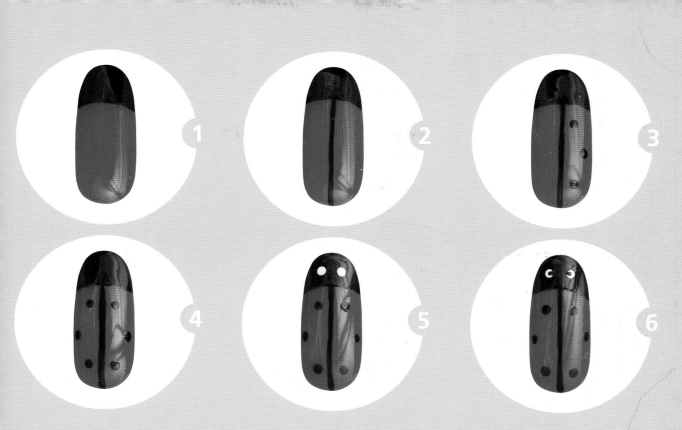

STEP 1

Apply a base coat to the nails and let it dry. Apply two coats of red nail polish and let it dry completely. Dip the thin nail art brush into the black nail polish and draw a horizontal line at the top third of the nail on the ring finger. Fill in the area from the line to the tip of the nail with black nail polish.

STEP 2

Draw a vertical line down the middle of the nail, from the base until the tip.

STEP 3

Dip the large dotting tool into the black nail polish and draw three evenly spaced dots on the right side of the middle line. The top and bottom dots should be closer to the middle line and the middle dot should be closer to the edge.

STEP 4

Draw three similar dots on the left side of the middle line. Try to make these dots mirror images of the dots on the right side of the line.

STEP 5

Clean the large dotting tool thoroughly and then dip it into the opaque white nail polish. Draw two dots in the black area at the tip of the nail for eyes.

STEP 6

Dip the small dotting tool into the black nail polish and draw a black dot on each white dot to finish the eyes. Decorate the rest of the nails by drawing evenly spaced black dots using the large dotting tool.

TIPS

• Wait until the polish is completely dry and then apply a top coat to seal and protect the design.
• Refresh the top coat regularly to keep the design looking fresh.

LEAPIN' LEOPARDS

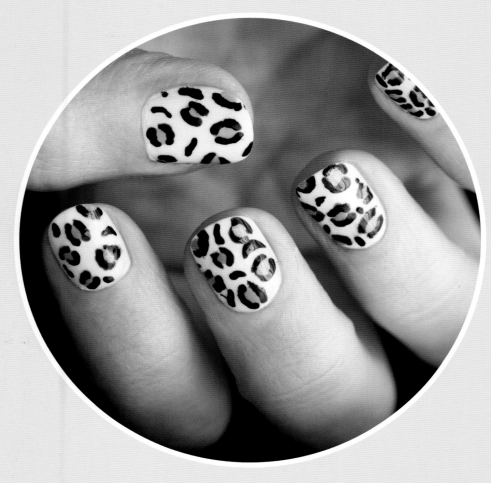

Is there a better way of completing an animal print outfit than with nails that match?

MATERIALS

For the Base:
- Opaque white nail polish

For the Design:
- Beige nail polish
- Black nail polish

TOOLS

- Thin nail art brush
- Dotting tool

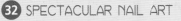

1

2

3

4

5

STEP 1

Apply a base coat to the nails and let it dry. Apply two coats of opaque white nail polish and let it dry completely. Using the beige nail polish, draw small dots on the nail. The dots don't need to be round and they shouldn't be identical either. Making each one a bit different adds to the authenticity of the design.

STEP 2

Dip the thin nail art brush into the black nail polish and draw two rounded lines around one of the dots. Like the dots, these lines don't need to be perfectly rounded. Leave a space between them so that they don't quite connect.

STEP 3

Repeat this step to draw rounded lines on either side of each dot.

STEP 4

Dip the dotting tool into the black nail polish and make a few dots on the nail in the white space between the beige dots.

STEP 5

Using the thin nail art brush, draw a few curved lines in the white space on the nail. Repeat these steps to make animal prints on all the nails.

TIPS

• Wait until the nails are completely dry and then apply a top coat to seal and protect the design.
• Refresh the top coat regularly to keep the design looking fresh.

ZEBRA ZAZING

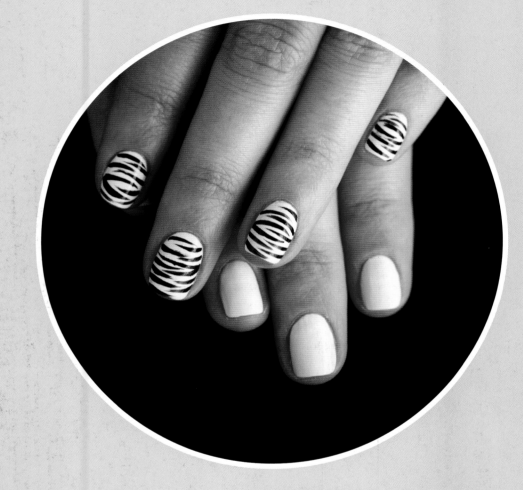

Add some zing to any black and white outfit with this wild design.

MATERIALS

For the Base:
- Opaque white nail polish

For the Design:
- Black nail polish

TOOLS
- Thin nail art brush

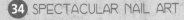

STEP 1
Apply a base coat to the nails and let it dry. Apply two coats of opaque white nail polish and let it dry completely.

STEP 2
Dip the thin nail art brush into the black nail polish and draw a single curved line that starts at the middle left edge of the nail and ends just past the middle of the nail. Make the line in a single stroke, and without using too much nail polish so it isn't too thick. The line should curve upwards and be thickest at the middle.

STEP 3
Draw a second line that starts at almost the same place at the right edge of the nail, curves above the first curved line, and ends near the left edge of the nail. The line should be similar in length and width to the first line, but it doesn't need to be identical.

STEP 4
Make a third curved line, similar to the first one, but a bit above it. Make sure there are thin strips of white space between each line. Make a fourth curved line that is similar to the first one but curves downwards rather than upwards.

STEP 5
Continue to make more curved lines, curving downwards on the bottom half of the nail and upwards on the top half of the nail, until the nail is filled. Make sure you leave white spaces between each line. Repeat this process to make zebra stripes on all the nails.

TIPS
• Wait until the nails are completely dry and then apply a top coat to seal and protect the design.
• Refresh the top coat regularly to keep the design looking fresh.

SWEETEST STRAWBERRIES

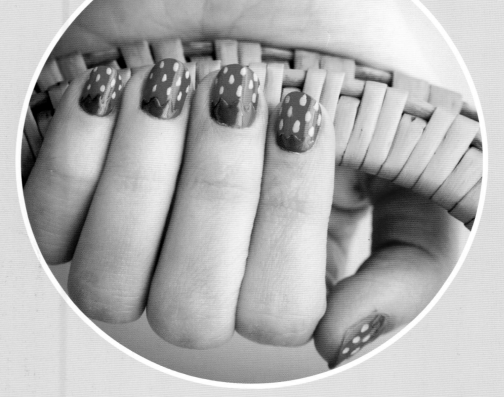

This design could have you wanting to nibble your nails,
so consider having a basket of fresh berries close by!

MATERIALS

For the Base:
• Red nail polish

For the Design:
• Green nail polish
• Yellow nail polish

TOOLS

• Toothpick
• Thin nail art brush

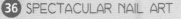

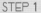

STEP 1

Apply a base coat to the nails and let it dry. Apply two coats of red nail polish and let it dry completely. Using a toothpick and the green nail polish, draw a horizontal zigzag line about one-third of the way up the nail from the base.

STEP 2

Using the thin art nail brush and the green nail polish, fill in the area between the base of the nail and the zigzag line. If you have a steady hand, you can use the regular nail polish brush to do this.

STEP 3

Clean the toothpick (or just use a new one) and dip it into the yellow nail polish. Draw three or four small lines above the zigzag green area. If you like, make small teardrop shapes instead of lines, with the tip of the teardrop facing the tip of the nail.

STEP 4

Draw a similar row of yellow lines or teardrops above this row, placing them in the intervals between yellow lines or teardrops of the first row.

STEP 5

Repeat this process to make a third row of lines or teardrops. Repeat all these steps to make strawberries on all the nails.

TIPS

• Wait until the nails are completely dry and then apply a top coat to seal and protect the design.
• Refresh the top coat regularly to keep the design looking fresh.

MUST-HAVE MUSTACHE

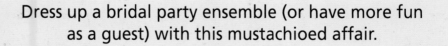

Dress up a bridal party ensemble (or have more fun
as a guest) with this mustachioed affair.

MATERIALS

For the Base:
- Turquoise nail polish

For the Design:
- Black nail polish

TOOLS

- Medium dotting tool
- Small dotting tool or toothpick

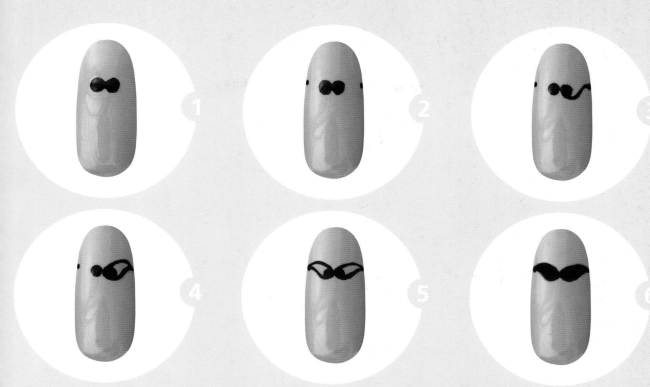

STEP 1
Apply a base coat to the nails and let it dry. Apply two coats of turquoise nail polish and let it dry completely. Dip the medium dotting tool into the black nail polish and draw two dots that touch each other near the top third of the nail.

STEP 2
Using the small dotting tool or toothpick, draw a dot on each side of the nail, a bit higher than the original two dots and very close to the edges.

STEP 3
Draw a curved line that connects the little dot at the right edge of the nail to the rightmost dot in the middle of the nail. The line should curve downwards just after it starts and then curve under the bottom of the rightmost middle dot.

STEP 4
Draw another curved line starting at the same little dot at the right edge of the nail. This line should curve upwards just after it starts and then curve over the top of the rightmost middle dot.

STEP 5
Repeat steps 3 and 4 on the other side of the nail.

STEP 6
Fill in the curved teardrops you have made on either side of the nail, using the small dotting tool or toothpick. Repeat these steps to make mustaches on all the nails. Alternately, you could decorate just one nail on each hand with a mustache.

TIPS
• Wait until the nails are completely dry and then apply a top coat to seal and protect the design.
• Refresh the top coat regularly to keep the design looking fresh.

GOLDEN HEARTS

This elegant design is both classy and trendy.
If you're short on time, skip the black outline.

MATERIALS

For the Base:
• Opaque white nail polish

For the Design:
• Gold nail polish
• Black nail polish

TOOLS

• Small dotting tool or toothpick
• Thin nail art brush

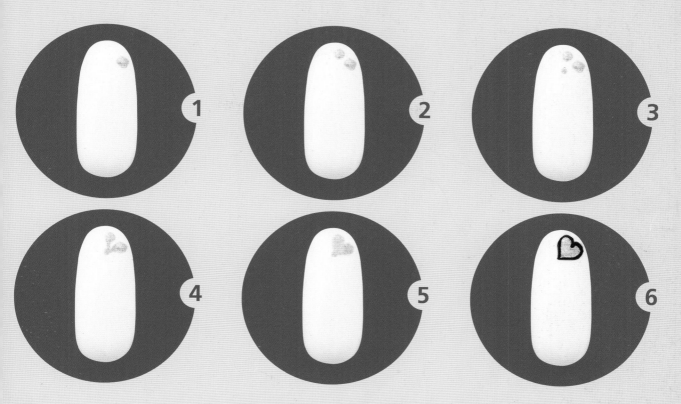

STEP 1
Apply a base coat to the nails and let it dry. Apply two coats of opaque white nail polish and let it dry completely. Dip the small dotting tool or toothpick into the gold nail polish and make a small plump dot near the top right corner of the nail.

STEP 2
Dip the dotting tool into the gold nail polish again and make a second plump dot, upwards and to the left a bit, of the first one.

STEP 3
Use the toothpick to draw a smaller dot below the second dot and a bit to the left to form a triangle of dots near the top right corner of the nail. The third dot

should be much smaller than the first two. It will be the tip of the heart.

STEP 4
Using the dotting tool or the toothpick to draw the nail polish from the rightmost dot diagonally towards the third dot to make the tip of the heart.

STEP 5
Repeat this technique with the second dot, drawing the polish towards the small dot you made in step 3 to complete the heart shape.

STEP 6
Wait for about 15 minutes until the nail polish is completely dry and then dip the thin nail art brush into

the black nail polish and draw a thin line around the golden heart. Repeat these steps to make golden hearts on all the nails.

TIPS
• Wait until the nails are completely dry and then apply a top coat to seal and protect the design.
• Refresh the top coat regularly to keep the design looking fresh.
• If you are worried about ruining the golden heart by drawing the black outline, omit this step and leave the golden heart as it is.

TUX DELUXE

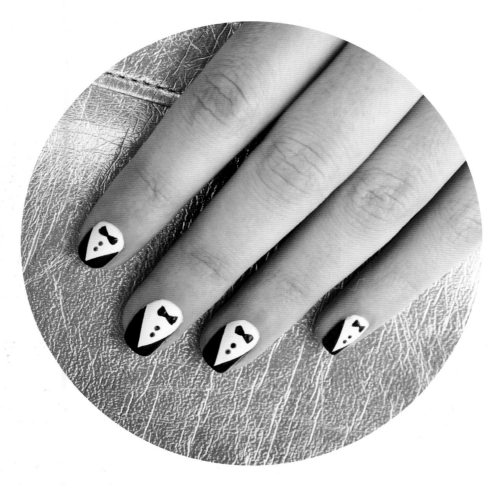

Why wait for a black-tie affair when you can wear
your tuxedo right on your nails?

MATERIALS

For the Base:
• Opaque white nail polish

For the Design:
• Black nail polish

TOOLS
• Thin nail art brush
• Small dotting tool

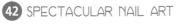

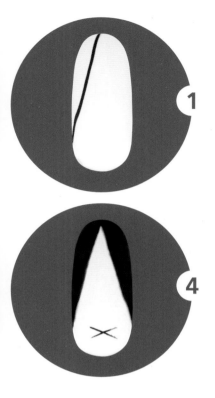

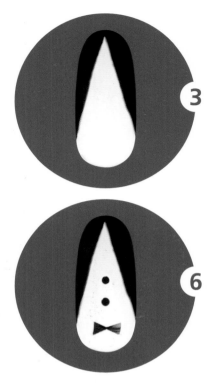

STEP 1
Apply a base coat to the nails and let it dry. Apply two coats of opaque white nail polish and let it dry completely. Dip the thin nail art brush into the black nail polish and draw a thin diagonal line that starts at the middle of the tip of the nail and ends on the left side of the nail, near the base.

STEP 2
Draw another thin line, similar in width and length, starting at the middle of the tip of the nail and ending on the right side of the nail, near the base. Try to make the two lines symmetrical.

STEP 3
Fill in the space between each line and the edge of the nail with black nail polish. You can use the thin nail art brush or the regular nail polish brush for this.

STEP 4
Draw a small X shape in the middle of the nail, close to the base but not touching it. This X should be wider than it is long, and shouldn't touch the lines you drew previously.

STEP 5
Using the thin nail art brush, fill in the right and left sides of the X to make the bowtie.

STEP 6
Dip the small dotting tool into the black nail polish and make two small dots, one above the other, along the middle of the nail. These are the buttons. Repeat these steps to make tuxedos on all the nails.

TIPS
• Wait until the nails are completely dry and then apply a top coat to seal and protect the design.
• Refresh the top coat regularly to keep the design looking fresh.

ROYAL RIBBONS

Upgrade a standard French manicure with a pretty bow.
Easy to do and full of "Wow"!

MATERIALS

For the Base:
- Light pink nail polish

For the Design:
- Opaque white nail polish
- Black nail polish
- Sparkly silver nail polish

TOOLS
- Thin nail art brush
- Small dotting tool or toothpick

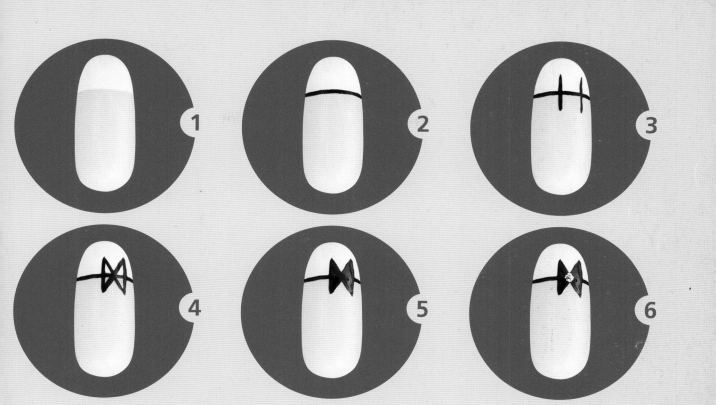

STEP 1

Apply a base coat to the nails and let it dry. Apply two coats of light pink nail polish and let it dry completely. Dip the thin nail art brush into the opaque white nail polish and draw a thick white line horizontally along the tip of the nail, much as you would in a French manicure. Fill in the tip of the nail with white nail polish. Wait for about 30 minutes, until the nail polish is completely dry.

STEP 2

Clean the thin nail art brush thoroughly, and then dip it into the black nail polish. Draw a thin line at the border between the white nail polish at the tip of the nail and the light pink nail polish on the base.

STEP 3

Draw two short vertical lines perpendicular to the black line you just drew. The first line should be at the middle of the nail and the second one should be halfway between the middle of the nail and the right edge.

STEP 4

Draw an X shape between these two short vertical lines.

STEP 5

Fill in the left and right side of the X shape with black nail polish to make a bow.

STEP 6

Dip the small dotting tool or toothpick into the silver nail polish and make a single dot in the middle of the bow. Repeat these steps to make bows on all the nails.

TIPS

• Wait until the nails are completely dry and then apply a top coat to seal and protect the design.
• Refresh the top coat regularly to keep the design looking fresh.

FRENCH TWIST

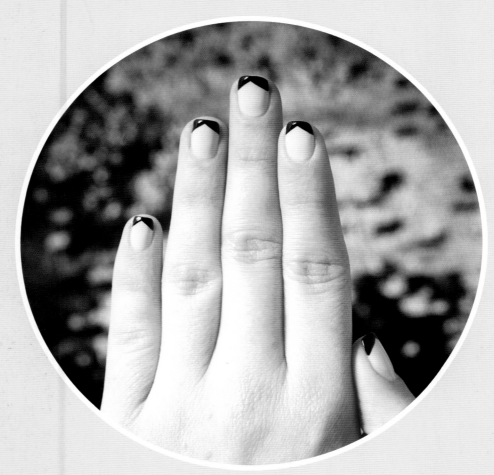

This design is an awesome and edgy twist on a traditional French manicure.

MATERIALS

For the Base:

• Opaque light pink nail polish

For the Design:

• Black nail polish

TOOLS

• Thin nail art brush

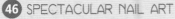

STEP 1
Apply a base coat to the nails and let it dry. Apply two coats of opaque light pink nail polish and let the polish dry.

STEP 2
Dip the thin nail art brush into the black nail polish and draw a diagonal line that starts at the right edge of the nail, about ¾ of the way up from the base, and ends at the tip of the nail, on the left side.

STEP 3
Draw a second diagonal line, this one starting about ¾ of the way up from the base on the left edge of the nail, and extending to the middle of the line that you made in step 2.

STEP 4
Fill in the two triangular shapes you made in steps 2 and 3 with black nail polish. Repeat these steps to make black tips on all the nails.

TIPS
• Wait until the nails are completely dry and then apply a top coat to seal and protect the design.
• Refresh the top coat regularly to keep the design looking fresh.

PEARLY BUBBLES

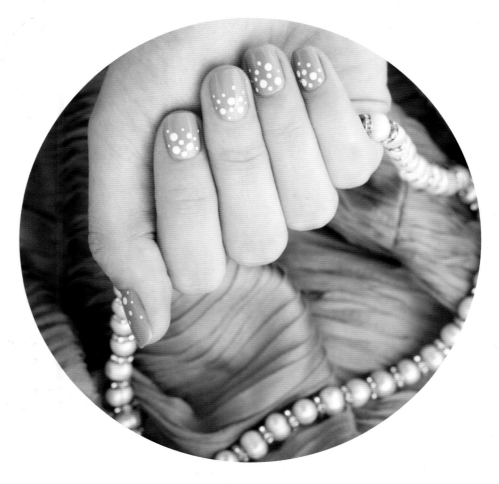

The secret to making successful bubbles is in the placement of the dots.

MATERIALS

For the Base:
- Opaque beige nail polish

For the Design:
- Opaque white nail polish

TOOLS

- Large dotting tool
- Medium dotting tool
- Small dotting tool or toothpick

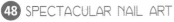

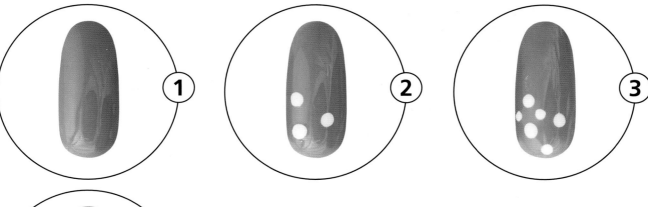

STEP 1

Apply a base coat to the nails and let it dry. Apply two coats of opaque beige nail polish and let it dry completely.

STEP 2

Dip the large dotting tool into the opaque white nail polish and make three scattered dots near the base of the nail. The dots should not go beyond the bottom half of the nail.

STEP 3

Use the medium dotting tool to make a few medium-sized dots interspersed between the larger dots. As before, these dots should remain in the bottom half of the nail.

STEP 4

Use the small dotting tool or toothpick to add a few more dots, interspersed amongst the medium and large dots, on the bottom half of the nail. Leave the tops of the nail dot-free and make sure none of the dots touch each other. Repeat these steps to make bubbly designs on all the nails.

TIPS

• Wait until the polish is completely dry and then apply a top coat to seal and protect the design.
• Refresh the top coat regularly to keep the design looking fresh.

CASCADING BLOSSOMS

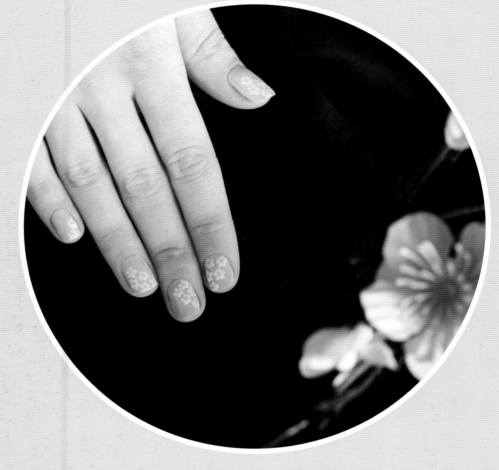

If you're in the mood for a delicate design, what could be gentler than a pretty cascade of tiny flowers?

MATERIALS

For the Base:
• Opaque light pink nail polish

For the Design:
• Opaque white nail polish

TOOLS
• Small dotting tool

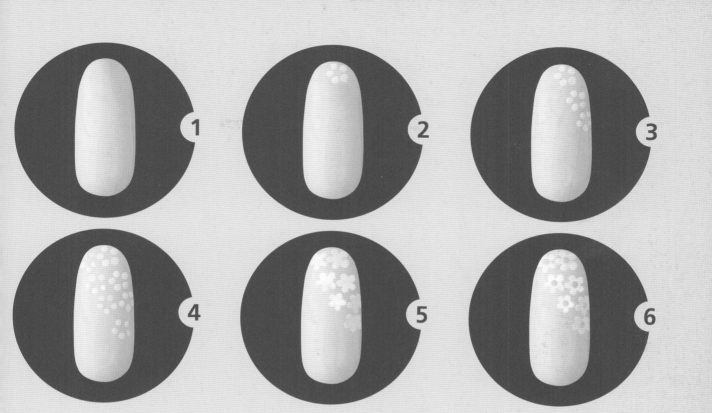

STEP 1
Apply a base coat to the nails and let it dry. Apply two coats of opaque light pink nail polish and let it dry completely.

STEP 2
Dip the dotting tool into the opaque white nail polish and make a cluster of five dots at the middle of the nail and near the tip, to make the petals for one flower.

STEP 3
Make a second cluster of dots in the same way, placing them a bit below the first cluster and closer to the right edge of the nail. Repeat this process to make a third cluster of dots, below the second cluster and quite close to the right edge of the nail. In this manner you'll create a 3-flower cascade.

STEP 4
Now make another cascading line of small flowers, immediately to the left of this one and containing 4 flowers. The first flower in this cascade should be placed at the tip of the nail, to the left of the first flower that you made in step 2.

STEP·5
Use the dotting tool to fill in the space in each flower with white nail polish.

STEP 6
Clean the dotting tool thoroughly and then dip it into the light pink nail polish that you used for the base. Make a single dot in the middle of each flower for the center. Repeat these steps to make cascading flowers on all the nails.

TIPS
• Wait until the polish is completely dry and then apply a top coat to seal and protect the design.
• Refresh the top coat regularly to keep the design looking fresh.

CHARMING CHICKADEES

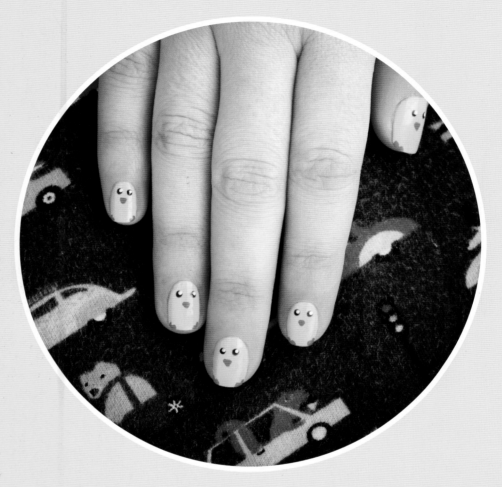

Add some charm to your life with these bright chickadees.

MATERIALS

For the Base:
- Yellow nail polish

For the Design:
- Orange nail polish
- Black nail polish
- Opaque white nail polish

TOOLS
- Small dotting tool or toothpick
- Large dotting tool

STEP 1
Apply a base coat to the nails and let it dry. Apply two coats of yellow nail polish and let it dry completely.

STEP 2
Dip the small dotting tool or toothpick into the orange nail polish and make a small triangle in the middle of the nail. The tip of the triangular should be at the middle of the nail and pointing towards the tip of the nail. This will be the chickadee's nose.

STEP 3
Dip the large dotting tool into the black nail polish and make two

small dots, one beside the other, between the triangle and the base of the nail. These will be the chickadee's eyes.

STEP 4
Dip the small dotting tool into the opaque white nail polish and make two small white dots on the black dots, to finish the eyes.

STEP 5
Clean the small dotting tool (or use a new toothpick) and dip it into the orange nail polish. Make a small semicircle at the tip of the nail and on the left side. This will be the chickadee's foot.

STEP 6
Make a second foot on the right side of the nail tip to complete the chickadee. Repeat these steps to make chickadees on all the nails.

TIPS
• Wait until the polish is completely dry and then apply a top coat to seal and protect the design.
• Refresh the top coat regularly to keep the design looking fresh.

PLAYFUL PENGUINS

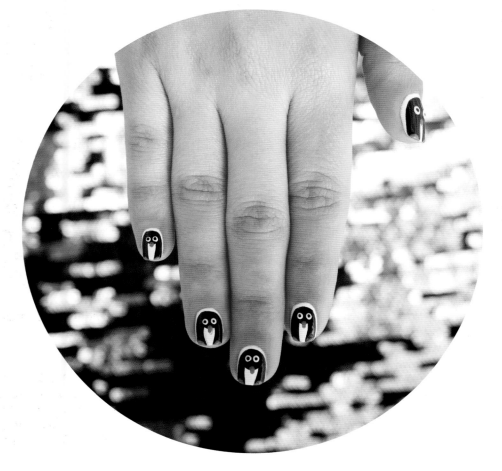

Why travel to the South Pole when you can create playful penguins right on your nails?

MATERIALS

For the Base:
- Opaque white nail polish

For the Design:
- Black nail polish
- Orange nail polish

TOOLS

- Large dotting tool
- Small dotting tool
- Toothpick

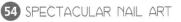

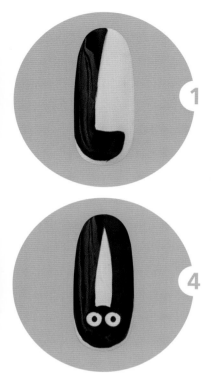

STEP 1

Apply a base coat to the nails and let it dry. Apply two coats of opaque white nail polish and let it dry completely. With the black nail polish, draw a thick line along the left edge of the nail, close to the edge but not quite touching it. The line should extend up to the middle of the tip of the nail. Draw a thick horizontal line across the base of the nail, also close to the edge but not touching it. Leaving a thin white line along the outer edge of the nail helps make the penguin image stand out.

STEP 2

Draw a thick line along the right side of the nail, similar to the line you drew at the beginning of step 1. The lines should meet at the middle tip of the nail to finish the penguin body.

STEP 3

Dip the large dotting tool into the white nail polish and make two dots on the black strip near the base of the nail, for the eyes.

STEP 4

Dip the small dotting tool into the black nail polish and make two smaller dots inside the larger white dots, to complete the eyes.

STEP 5

Dip a toothpick into the orange nail polish and make one tiny triangle below the eyes, to make the beak. The tip of the triangle should point towards the tip of the nail.

STEP 6

Dip a toothpick into the orange nail polish and make two tiny semicircles at the edge of the nail, for feet. Repeat these steps to make perfect little penguins on all the nails.

TIPS

• Wait until the polish is completely dry and then apply a top coat to seal and protect the design.
• Refresh the top coat regularly to keep the design looking fresh.

 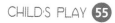

DOGGIE PAWS

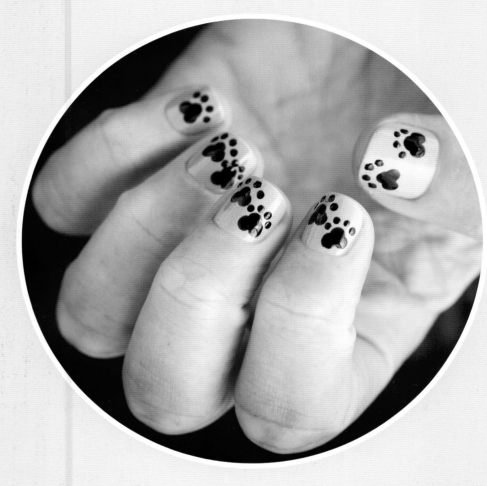

If you love dogs, your paws will be delighted to be decorated with these ones!

MATERIALS

For the Base:
• Lavender nail polish

For the Design:
• Black nail polish

TOOLS
• Large dotting tool
• Small dotting tool or toothpick

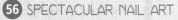

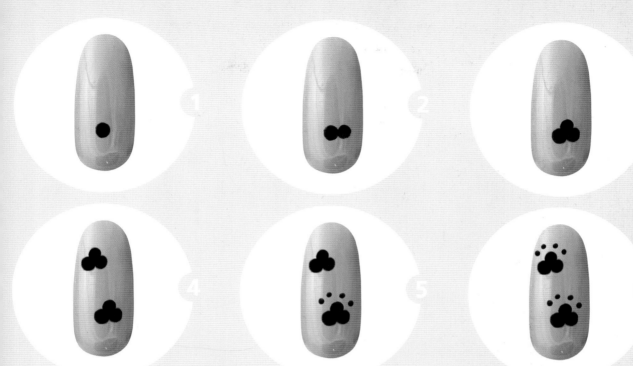

STEP 1

Apply a base coat to the nails and let it dry. Apply two coats of lavender nail polish and let it dry completely. Dip the large dotting tool into the black nail polish and make a large dot at the middle of the nail, near the base.

STEP 2

Make another large dot, right beside the first dot and touching it.

STEP 3

Make a third dot just above the first two dots and touching both of them. This dot should join the other two dots together to create a paw shape.

STEP 4

Repeat these steps to make another trio of dots elsewhere on the nail.

STEP 5

Dip the small dotting tool or toothpick into the black nail polish and make a curved line of four dots above the first paw.

STEP 6

Repeat this step to make four dots above the other paw. Repeat this process to make paws on all the nails. Adjust the number of paws you make according to the size of the nail.

TIPS

• Wait until the polish is completely dry and then apply a top coat to seal and protect the design.
• Refresh the top coat regularly to keep the design looking fresh.

PUFFY CLOUDS

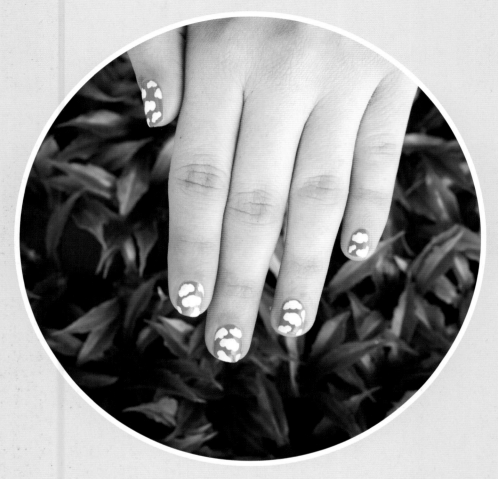

Whatever the weather, enjoy picture-perfect skies with this pretty design.

MATERIALS

For the Base:
• Light blue nail polish

For the Design:
• Opaque white nail polish

TOOLS

• Large dotting tool

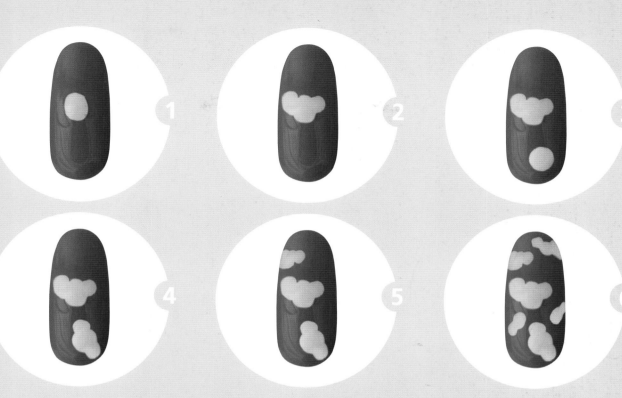

STEP 1

Apply a base coat to the nails and let it dry. Apply two coats of light blue nail polish and let it dry completely. Dip the large dotting tool into the opaque white nail polish and make a plump dot at the middle of the nail.

STEP 2

Make two more dots, on the right and left side of the first dot and touching it. The dots should be placed slightly above or below the first dot, and should be slightly different in size, to create a nice irregular shape that looks cloud-like.

STEP 3

Make another plump dot near the base of the nail.

STEP 4

Add a few more dots, much in the same way as you did in step 2, to make a second cloud shape.

STEP 5

Repeat this process to make a third cloud near the tip of the nail. You don't need to make an entire cloud – even a partial one is great.

STEP 6

Repeat these steps to make a few more clouds on this nail, and all the other nails. Adjust the number of clouds you make on each nail, according to the size of the nail.

TIPS

• Wait until the polish is completely dry and then apply a top coat to seal and protect the design.
• Refresh the top coat regularly to keep the design looking fresh.

PUZZLE PIECES

This design is a perfect fit for puzzle fanatics of any age.
Best of all – you'll never lose any pieces!

MATERIALS

For the Base:
- Yellow nail polish
- Turquoise nail polish

For the Design:
- Fuchsia nail polish
- Green nail polish

TOOLS
- Small dotting tool or toothpick

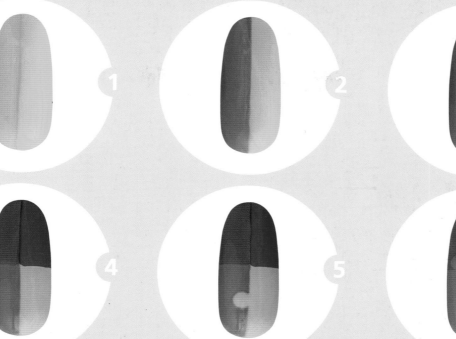

STEP 1
Apply a base coat to the nails and let it dry. Apply two coats of yellow nail polish on the right half of the nail and let it dry completely.

STEP 2
Apply two coats of turquoise nail polish on the left half of the nail and let it dry completely.

STEP 3
Apply two coats of fuchsia nail polish on the top half of the yellow half of the nail.

STEP 4
Apply two coats of green nail polish on the top half of the turquoise half of the nail.

STEP 5
Dip the small dotting tool or toothpick into the yellow nail polish and make a small yellow dot on the turquoise quarter of the nail, in the middle of the border between the yellow and the turquoise quarter. Make sure the dot touches the yellow quarter.

STEP 6
Repeat this process with the other colors, making a turquoise dot on the green quarter, at the middle of the border between the green and turquoise quarters, a green dot on the fuchsia quarter, at the middle of the border between the fuchsia and green quarters, and a fuchsia dot on the yellow quarter, at the middle of the border between the yellow and fuchsia quarters. Make sure all of the dots touch the adjacent quarter so that they look connected. Repeat these steps to make puzzle pieces on all the nails.

TIPS
• Wait until the polish is completely dry and then apply a top coat to seal and protect the design.
• Refresh the top coat regularly to keep the design looking fresh.
• If you're having trouble making straight lines for each quarter, try using a bit of adhesive tape. For tips on using adhesive tape, see page 9.

CHERRY ⊙N TOP

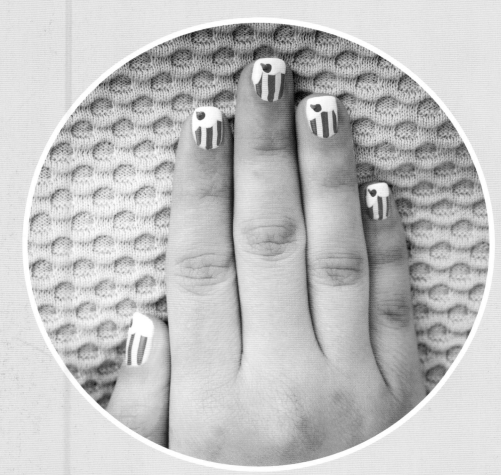

Guilt-free ice cream, complete with whipped cream and a cherry on top. Yum!

MATERIALS

For the Base:
• Opaque light pink nail polish

For the Design:
• Fuchsia nail polish
• Opaque white nail polish
• Red nail polish
• Green nail polish

TOOLS
• Thin nail art brush
• Small dotting tool or toothpick
• Toothpick

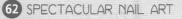

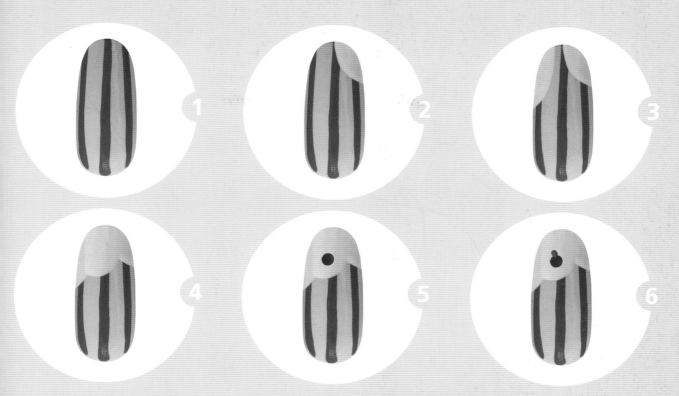

STEP 1

Apply a base coat to the nails and let it dry. Apply two coats of opaque light pink nail polish and let it dry completely. Dip the thin nail art brush into the fuchsia nail polish and draw a line down the middle of the nail, from the base to the tip. Make two more lines, one on either side of this middle line; the lines should be similar in width. Let the nail polish dry for about 15 minutes.

STEP 2

Dip the regular nail polish brush into the opaque white nail polish and make a semicircle on the right side of the nail tip, for the whipped cream.

STEP 3

Make a second semicircle on the left side of the nail, starting at the tip and extending downwards. This semi-circle should be a bit longer than the first one.

STEP 4

Make a third semicircle at the middle tip of the. This semicircle should overlap with the first two semicircles to complete the whipped cream. Let the nail polish dry for about 15 minutes.

STEP 5

Dip the small dotting tool into the red nail polish and make a single dot on the white area, for the cherry.

STEP 6

Dip the thin nail art brush into the green nail polish and make a small line on top of the cherry, for the stem. Repeat these steps to make whipped cream-topped sundaes on all the nails.

TIPS

• Wait until the polish is completely dry and then apply a top coat to seal and protect the design.
• Refresh the top coat regularly to keep the design looking fresh.

BUMBLING BEAUTIES

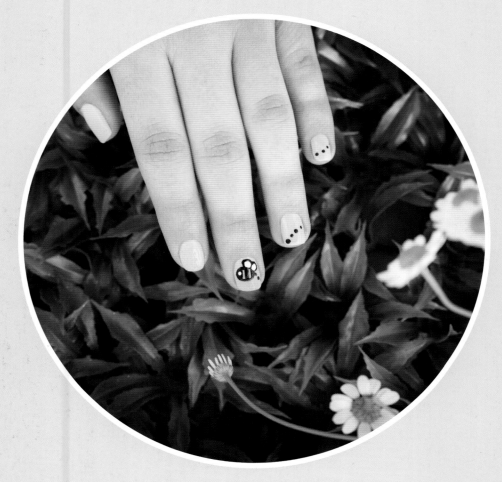

Your nails will buzz with glee after being decorating with these adorable bees.

MATERIALS

For the Base:
- Yellow nail polish

For the Design:
- Black nail polish
- Opaque white nail polish

TOOLS
- Thin nail art brush
- Small dotting tool or toothpick

STEP 1
Apply a base coat to the nails and let it dry. Apply two coats of yellow nail polish and let it dry completely. With the thin nail art brush and the black nail polish, draw the outline of an oval shape in the middle of the nail on the index finger. This will be the bee's body.

STEP 2
Draw three thick black vertical lines inside the oval shape. The black lines should be more or less the same thickness as the space between the lines.

STEP 3
Still using the black nail polish, draw two little circles along the bottom of the oval and closer to the left side, for the wings.

STEP 4
Draw a tiny horizontal line extending from the left side of the bee's body, for the stinger.

STEP 5
Dip the small dotting tool or toothpick into the opaque white nail polish and fill in the wings. Use the white nail polish to make a small dot at the right side of the bee's body, for the eye.

STEP 6
Dip the small dotting tool into the black nail polish and make several tiny dots trailing from the stinger, to show the bee's path. Continue this path of dots on the nails of the ring finger and little finger. Repeat this entire process on the other hand.

TIPS
• Wait until the polish is completely dry and then apply a top coat to seal and protect the design.
• Refresh the top coat regularly to keep the design looking fresh.

RETRO DOTS

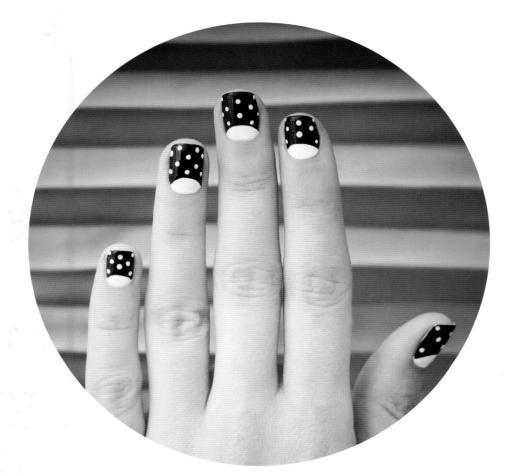

Add some funk to a traditional half-moon manicure with frolicking fun polka dots.

MATERIALS

For the Base:
- Opaque white nail polish

For the Design:
- Black nail polish

TOOLS
- Round stickers
- Small dotting tool or toothpick

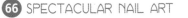

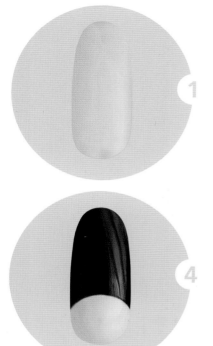

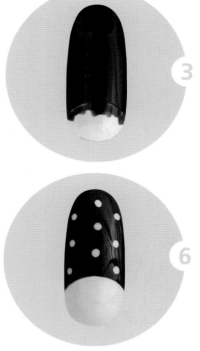

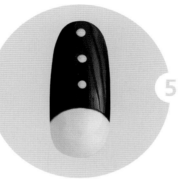

STEP 1
Apply a base coat to the nails and let it dry. Apply two coats of opaque white nail polish and let it dry for about 30 minutes. Because you'll be using stickers in the next step, make sure the nail polish is completely dry before you continue.

STEP 2
Place a round sticker on your hand (not yet on your nail) and pull it off. Repeat this action a few times to reduce the stickiness of the sticker. You want the sticker to stick to the nail, but not stick too well. Place the sticker at the base of the nail, adjusting it so that it creates a symmetrical semicircle shape at the base of the nail.

STEP 3
Apply two coats of black nail polish to the nail. Paint over the edge of the sticker but don't allow the polish to go to the base of the nail. (If the sticker has a hole in it, like the one I've chosen, make sure you don't paint the area of the nail that's exposed in the hole.)

STEP 4
Wait for about 30 seconds and then carefully remove the sticker. Peel the sticker backwards, rather than upwards, to make sure you don't smudge the polish.

STEP 5
Dip the small dotting tool or toothpick into the opaque white nail polish and make three evenly spaced dots in a vertical line along the middle of the nail.

STEP 6
Make two more vertical lines of dots on the nail, one on each side of the first line of dots. These dots should be placed at the intervals between the dots in the first line. Repeat these steps to make semicircles and dots on all the nails.

TIPS
• Wait until the polish is completely dry and then apply a top coat to seal and protect the design.
• Refresh the top coat regularly to keep the design looking fresh.

SUPER SIMPLE STRIPES

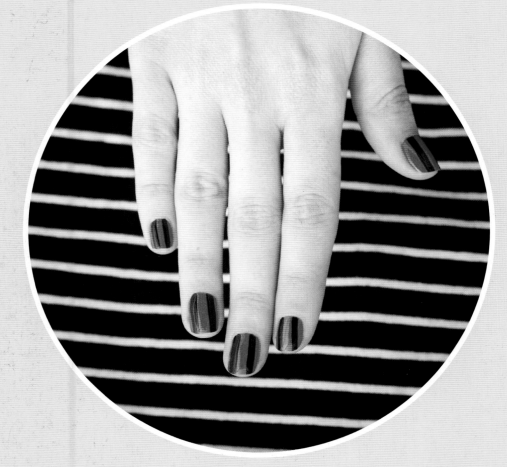

Guess what! You don't need any special skills to create perfect stripes on your nails. Just two colors of nail polish and a few strips of tape.

MATERIALS

For the Base:
- Fuchsia nail polish

For the Design:
- Black nail polish

TOOLS
- Adhesive tape
- Scissors

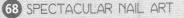

STEP 1

Apply a base coat to the nails and let it dry. Apply two coats of fuchsia nail polish and let it dry for about 30 minutes. Because you'll be using tape in the next step, make sure the nail polish is completely dry before you continue.

STEP 2

Place a few pieces of adhesive tape on your hand (not yet on your nail) and pull them off. Repeat this action a few times to reduce the stickiness of the tape. You want the tape to stick to the nail, but not stick too well. Place three strips of tape vertically on a nail, at even intervals.

STEP 3

Apply two coats of black nail polish to the nail.

STEP 4

Wait for about 30 seconds and then carefully pull off the tape. Make sure you pull the tape backwards, rather than upwards, to avoid smudging the nail polish. Repeat these steps to make stripes on all the nails.

TIPS

• Wait until the polish is completely dry and then apply a top coat to seal and protect the design.
• Refresh the top coat regularly to keep the design looking fresh.
• To prepare for this design, cut several thin strips of tape, even in width, and keep them close at hand. For tips on using adhesive tape, see page 9.

CHIC CHECKS

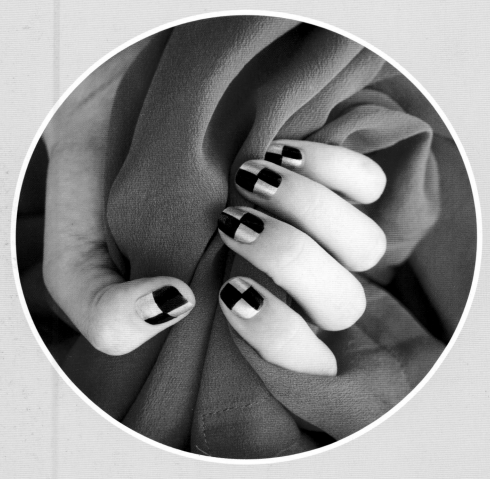

Here's an easy way to make tidy checkerboards on your nails.
Maximum effect; minimum effort!

MATERIALS

For the Base:
• Gold nail polish

For the Design:
• Black nail polish

TOOLS
• Adhesive tape
• Scissors

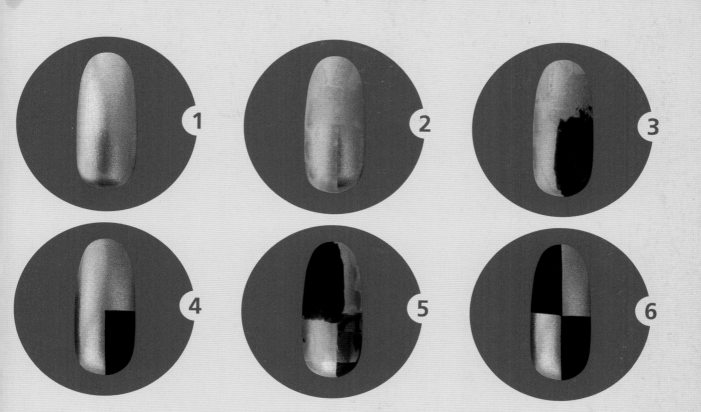

STEP 1
Apply a base coat to the nails and let it dry. Apply two coats of gold nail polish and let it dry for about 30 minutes. Because you'll be using tape in the next step, make sure the nail polish is completely dry before you continue.

STEP 2
Place two pieces of adhesive tape on your hand (not yet on your nail) and pull them off. Repeat this action a few times to reduce the stickiness of the tape. You want the tape to stick to the nail, but not stick too well. Place one piece of tape lengthwise along the left half of the nail. Place the other piece of tape widthwise along the top half of the nail.

STEP 3
Apply two coats of black nail polish to the exposed bottom right quarter of the nail. Allow the polish to go over the edge of the tape.

STEP 4
Wait for about 30 seconds and then carefully pull off the pieces of tape. Make sure you pull the tape backwards, rather than upwards, to avoid smudging the nail polish. Wait for about 30 minutes to allow the polish to dry completely.

STEP 5
Place two more pieces of tape on your hand and pull them off. Repeat this action a few times to reduce the stickiness of the tape. Place one piece of tape lengthwise along the right half of the nail and the other piece of tape widthwise along the bottom half of the nail. Apply two coats of black nail polish to the exposed quarter of the nail. Allow the polish to go over the edge of the tape.

STEP 6
Wait for about 30 seconds and then carefully pull off the pieces of tape. Make sure you pull the tape backwards, rather than upwards, to avoid smudging the nail polish. Repeat these steps to make checkerboards on all the nails.

TIPS
• Wait until the polish is completely dry and then apply a top coat to seal and protect the design.
• Refresh the top coat regularly to keep the design looking fresh.
• For tips on using adhesive tape, see page 9.

TRIANGULAR TRICKS

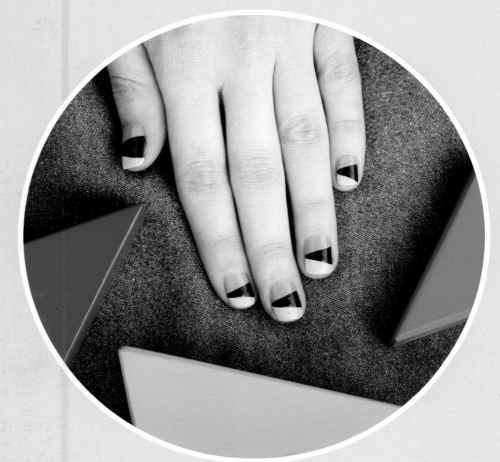

You don't have to like geometry to love this geometric design—classic, yet cool.

MATERIALS

For the Base:
- Beige nail polish

For the Design:
- Yellow nail polish
- Black nail polish

TOOLS
- Adhesive tape
- Scissors

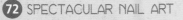

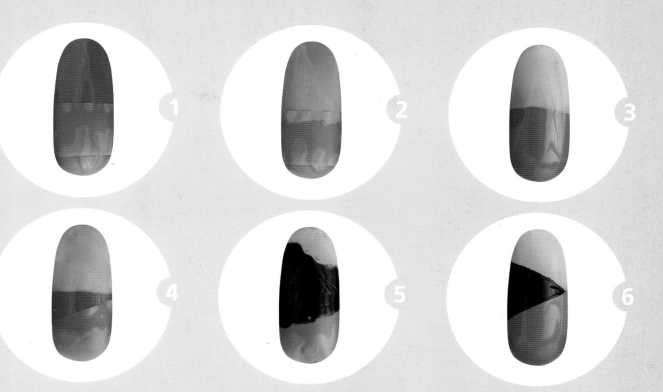

STEP 1

Apply a base coat to the nails and let it dry. Apply two coats of beige nail polish and let it dry for about 30 minutes. Because you'll be using tape in the next step, make sure the nail polish is completely dry before you continue. Place a piece of adhesive tape on your hand (not yet on your nail) and pull it off. Repeat this action a few times to reduce the stickiness of the tape. Place a piece of tape horizontally along the bottom half of the nail.

STEP 2

Apply two coats of yellow nail polish to the exposed top half of the nail. Paint the polish over the top edge of the tape.

STEP 3

Wait for about 30 seconds and

then carefully remove the tape. Peel the tape off backwards, rather than upwards, so that you don't smudge the polish. Let the polish dry for about 30 minutes. Because you'll be using tape again in the next step, make sure the yellow nail polish is completely dry before you continue.

STEP 4

Place two pieces of tape on your hand (not yet on your nail) and pull them off. Repeat this action a few times to reduce the stickiness of the tape. Place one piece of tape diagonally along the top of the nail and another piece of tape diagonally, in the opposite direction, along the bottom of the nail. Leave a bare, triangular shape in the middle of the nail that is half brown and half yellow.

STEP 5

Apply two coats of black nail polish to the exposed part of the nail. Paint the polish over the edges of tape.

STEP 6

Wait for about 30 seconds and then carefully remove the pieces of tape. Repeat these steps to make colorful triangles on all the nails.

TIPS

• Wait until the polish is completely dry and then apply a top coat to seal and protect the design.
• Refresh the top coat regularly to keep the design looking fresh.
• For tips on using adhesive tape, see page 9.

DISCO DELIGHT

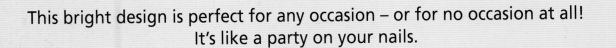

This bright design is perfect for any occasion – or for no occasion at all!
It's like a party on your nails.

MATERIALS

For the Base:
- Neon pink nail polish
- Neon yellow nail polish
- Neon green nail polish

For the Design:
- Black nail polish

TOOLS

- Extra thin nail stickers

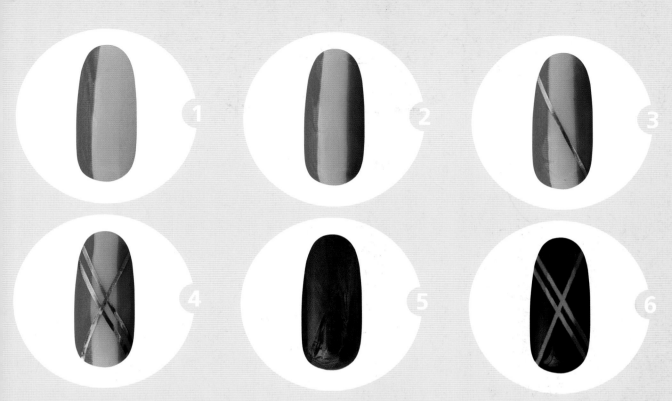

STEP 1

Apply a base coat to the nails and let it dry. Apply two coats of neon pink nail polish in a thick vertical strip that covers the left third of the nail. Apply two coats of neon yellow nail polish in a thick vertical strip along the middle third of the nail.

STEP 2

Apply two coats of neon green nail polish in a thick vertical strip along the remaining third of the nail. Let the polish dry for about 30 minutes. Because you'll be using stickers in the next step, make sure the nail polish is completely dry before you continue.

STEP 3

Place an extra thin nail sticker diagonally across the nail, from the green side of the nail near the base to the pink side of the nail, near the tip. Leave a small tail of the sticker extending from one end – you'll need this to pull off the sticker later.

STEP 4

Place a second sticker on the nail, parallel to and above the first sticker. Place a third sticker on the nail, diagonally and in the opposite direction, which extends from the pink side of the nail at the base to the green side of the nail near the tip.

STEP 5

Apply two coats of black nail polish on the entire nail.

STEP 6

Wait for about 30 seconds and then carefully remove all three stickers. Peel the stickers backwards, rather than upwards, so that you don't smudge the polish. Repeat these steps on all the nails. You can apply the stickers in different patterns on each nail or make them all the same.

TIPS

• Wait until the polish is completely dry and then apply a top coat to seal and protect the design.
• Refresh the top coat regularly to keep the design looking fresh.

AWESOMELY ARGYLE

Bring argyle to places it never imagined. Your nails will be the envy of sweaters everywhere!

MATERIALS

For the Base:
- Light purple nail polish

For the Design:
- Opaque light pink nail polish
- Opaque white nail polish

TOOLS
- Thin nail art brush

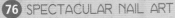

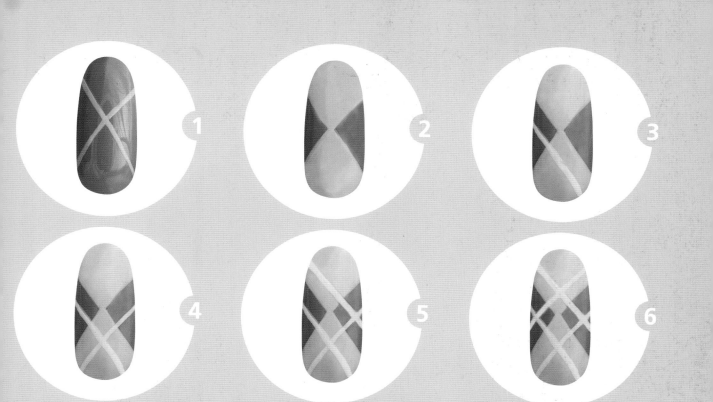

STEP 1
Apply a base coat to the nails and let it dry. Apply two coats of light purple nail polish and let it dry completely. Dip the thin nail art brush into the opaque light pink nail polish and make a large X on the nail.

STEP 2
Fill in the triangles that were formed by the X at the tip and the base of the nail with the opaque light pink nail polish and then let the polish dry for about 30 minutes.

STEP 3
Clean the thin nail art brush thoroughly and then dip it into the opaque white nail polish. Make a diagonal line that extends from the base of the nail on the right side to the edge of the nail on the left side, just above the middle of the nail. This line should be parallel to the line drawn in step 2 to make the original X shape.

STEP 4
Make a diagonal line in the opposite direction, from the base of the nail on the left side to the edge of the nail on the right side, just above the middle of the nail. This line should be parallel to the other line that formed the original X shape.

STEP 5
Make a third diagonal white line, parallel to the white line drawn in step 3, from the right edge of the nail, just below the middle, to the left side of the nail, near the tip.

STEP 6
Make one more diagonal white line, parallel to the white line drawn in step 4, from the right edge of the nail, just below the middle, to the left side of the nail, near the tip. Repeat these steps to make argyle designs on all the nails.

TIPS
• Wait until the polish is completely dry and then apply a top coat to seal and protect the design.
• Refresh the top coat regularly to keep the design looking fresh.

WAVY STRIPES

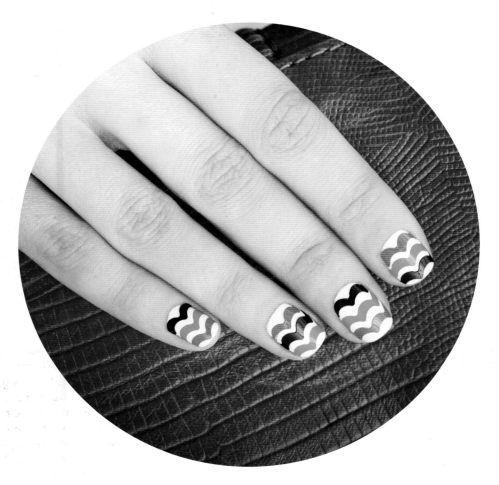

Here's an example of great nail art that requires no artistic skills at all—just some clever cutting and pasting!

MATERIALS

For the Base:
- Opaque white nail polish

For the Design:
- Orange nail polish
- Black nail polish
- Turquoise nail polish

TOOLS
- Adhesive tape
- Zigzag scissors

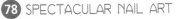

STEP 1
Apply a base coat to the nails and let it dry. Apply two coats of opaque white nail polish and let it dry completely.

STEP 2
Unroll a 4-inch piece of adhesive tape and paint patches of orange, black and turquoise nail polish on the tape. Let the polish on the tape dry completely and then cut the painted patches of tape into single-color strips using a zigzag scissors. The strips should be more or less even in width.

STEP 3
Affix an orange strip near the base of the nail.

STEP 4
Affix a turquoise strip above the orange strip. Leave a space between the two strips about the same width as the strips themselves, and try to line up the curves in the zigzag.

STEP 5
Affix a black strip above the turquoise strip, as you did in step 3.

STEP 6
If there is more room on the nail, affix more strips of painted tape. Repeat these steps on all the nails, altering the pattern of the colors if you like.

TIPS
• Apply a top coat over the strips of tape to affix them onto the nails and protect the design.
• Refresh the top coat regularly to keep the design looking fresh.
• For a different look that uses the same technique, adjust the space you leave between the strips or use different types of scissors to cut the strips.